Imagine
They Are Lonely Children

A Neuroscience Perspective on Development

John D. Hartman, MT-BC, NMT Fellow

WESTBOW
P R E S S®
A DIVISION OF THOMAS NELSON
& ZONDERVAN

WestBow Press books may be ordered through booksellers or by contacting:

WestBow Press
A Division of Thomas Nelson & Zondervan
1663 Liberty Drive
Bloomington, IN 47403
www.westbowpress.com
844-714-3454

Interior Image Credit: Andrew Neary, MT-BC, NMT

ISBN: 978-1-9736-6820-6 (sc)
ISBN: 978-1-9736-6821-3 (e)

Library of Congress Control Number: 2019911379

Print information available on the last page.

WestBow Press rev. date: 8/25/2020

Forward

To my God, my family and to the least of these, this is for you. This is my attempt to clear the fog and allow the bright rays of truth, hope and faith to shine in every life. Several simple but forgotten principles seem to have been lost and I hope to reinspire society with their glowing embers. All people are created equal. All people are created in God's image and He wants all of us to come to the knowledge of truth. What is truth? Is truth relevant or individually defined? Are there timeless principles that are undeniable? How has multiculturalism destroyed our melting pot and how do we refine that melting pot and begin the transformation that produces fruit radiant like gold? Does our great nation still offer this truth and hope to all, or do we just say so, not believing, promoting, and supporting every citizen? Is the answer because we don't know how or that we don't want to? If you are equipped with the tools to do so, will you use them in the face of great opposition? Will you join me in walking down this good and right path?

Acknowledgements

First and foremost, I thank God Almighty. You have guided me through dark valleys and blessed me beyond measure in countless ways. You allowed my sight to be taken from me at a young age, and have guided me on the narrow path, and given me the ability to pursue my dreams, the power to believe in my passion, and special vision for sharing the gifts you have blessed me with to serve others. I could never have completed this book without our relationship and the faith I have in you.

To my beautiful wife, Sherry, and my incredible children, you are the greatest blessing in my life. I am eternally grateful for your love and daily support. All the good that comes from this book, I look forward to sharing with you. Your sacrifices of our time together so that others may benefit, and for God's kingdom, is very appreciated. I love you always and forever!

To my educational and professional colleagues, your contributions to the fields of Music Therapy and Neurologic Music Therapy have provided a firm foundation to build upon. It has been my pleasure to learn from and work alongside so many of you. I am especially grateful to my friends and colleagues with Across the Way – Community Resource Center, Inc. Our philosophy of independence promotes both functional and financial self-sustaining freedom. Our developmental and reimbursement reduction plan and model is an excellent example of operational values based on God's word. Thank you for your dedication to transform the systems that perpetuate dependence, and for supporting professionals and programs that share these values. Your encouragement and support has helped make this book possible. It is my pleasure to pray with you and serve as God guides as we respect the dignity, uniqueness, and intrinsic value of every person. May God richly bless each of you and ATW-CRC in this journey.

I also need to offer special thanks and blessing to the individuals and their families who allowed me to use their personal stories in this book to offer hope and opportunity to many others who are struggling to reach their own potential and God-given purposes. It is on your behalf and for your futures I pray. I dream about outcomes and fulfillment for you while tirelessly working. It is your futures I aim to secure with joy, love and opportunity. For the privacy and protection of these consumers, their names have been changed, and the setting of their treatment concealed.

Finally, special thanks to Linda and Leanne for offering their time and talent to edit and review my manuscript. My chicken scratches and finger fumbles certainly were a challenge, but you persevered. Also thank you, Rob, for hosting me for a weekend of fun, memories and dedication, while applying final edits with the track changes. I pray that all of you are blessed in special ways for your love and support.

Matthew 25:40 (NIV)
The King will reply, "Truly I tell you, whatever you did for one of the least of these brothers and sisters of mine, you did for me."

Introduction

Two years ago, after almost 15 years of treating adults with developmental disabilities, I was asked to consider working with children. Children's programming represented a new division at my facility in the Midwest, and I said yes. After scrubbing my hands, I walked through the door of the childcare facility designed to serve the most severely impaired infants, toddlers, and children. Each child was unique, impaired from birth or gut-wrenching child abuse and trauma. Each child lay in a kid cart, or a beanbag sort of bed, or a prison barred safety crib. Buzzers blared warning beeps asserting urgency and need. The children cried out in reflexive utterances responding to the invasive lifesaving medical treatment. Why the need for such a program? Honestly, if the children weren't at this facility, they would be confined to a hospital or nursing facility.

As a music therapist, I wondered what to do next? Should I pull out my guitar and sing hello? Could I pass out the instruments to allow the children to play along with me? Sadly, I tried that, but unfortunately, it wasn't effective.

What does the special educator do? Would repetition and reinforcement work to teach basic cognitive concepts?

What does the traditional therapy team do? Well in this case, they completed the assessment to determine if the children qualify for reimbursable authorization. Unfortunately, these children do not generally progress quickly enough to warrant 8, 10 or 14 sessions to teach feeding, language, range of motion, or strength training therapy. In other words, prior authorization probably will not be approved.

Most clinicians have experienced these types of challenges from clients or children at some point in their careers, leaving them to continue to ask: "What to do next?"

Challenges emerge from the beginning. First, I needed to complete the clinical assessment, which turned out to be a major roadblock. The clinical assessment tool required the child identify and vocalize concepts like color and shape as well as demonstrate fine and gross motor skills. This proved impossible given these children were unaware of what they were hearing, seeing, or experiencing. They were unable to move or speak. They each achieved an extremely low score on the test, resulting in a rating of never or rarely achieving the skill. The truth is that the assessment failed to appropriately identify the problem underlying each child's disability. More frighteningly, however, the assessment concluded that these children would never acquire the skills allowing them to leave the facility and live an independent life.

The problem of assessment was difficult to untangle. How could anyone assess potential ability locked inside an unresponsive child? The neurologist had already assessed the children in the facility using the Glasgow Coma scale and most scored as a vegetative state (VS) or a minimally conscious state (MCS).

The next problem was the standard treatment options. In the school setting, traditionally a team of experts would develop an individualized education plan (IEP) for the child to develop the skills associated with learning colors, shapes, and fine and gross motor movement. The team would incorporate repetition, reinforcement, and redirection to assist the child in achieving the cognitive and age-related goals in the areas of reading, writing, and arithmetic. This model represents current best practices in the academic and clinical worlds. Even in a clinical setting, as in the one I describe, the staff members retain the cognitive goals of reading, writing, and arithmetic by adapting individualized approaches to achieve the goals for each child. The special education teacher may physically assist the child in a vegetative state to place his or her hand upon an object while verbally speaking the name of the object for the child.

This procedure achieves an age appropriate approach designed to teach the child to learn a concept. Yet, the children I served were diagnosed in a vegetative state, usually indicating that the children functioned without awareness of either the teacher or the object, and more importantly, were unable to reach the complex cognitive goals.

How can best practices become better? I turned to Neurologic Music Therapists who believed that certain individuals who were unable to respond to the environment, similar to some of the kids I served, were unresponsive because on the neurological level, they were unable to *initiate* a response (Guldenmund, Stender, Heine, & Laureys, 2012). Without initiating a response, the vegetative child remains motionless. Neurologic Music Therapy (NMT), a Transformational Design Model (TDM) based in neuroscience research, uses different assessments and treatment, and allowed for transition to independence for several of the children I served.

Let's take the problem of assessment

Briefly, the Glasgow Coma Scale accurately and reliably assesses the child's ability to respond cognitively to the environment. Four children with similar Glasgow Coma Scale scores of vegetative state could and probably do have four different neurological reasons for their disabilities and subsequent lack of response. Assessment requires identifying the unique neurological processes underpinning each individual's state.

Diagnostic differentiation allows the therapist to identify the specific neurologic needs of each individual, allowing the professional to identify which neurological processes need to be addressed and which specific neurologic stimulus affects those processes. The Transformational Design Model identifies the disrupted neurological processes and a clinician applies the correct neurological stimulus to affect that process. The Neurologic Music Therapist then builds a treatment protocol including stimulating a neurological sequence designed to drive the nervous system toward health.

Instead of using repetition, reinforcement, and redirection, the treatment involves a rhythmic auditory stimulus in the form of music, which serves to initiate neural activity, sustaining or inhibiting each neurological sequence or process. In this way, the diagnostic details define the treatment, which may include neurologic music therapists, and depending on the client, a variety of traditional therapists to implement the treatment. This process allowed me to create a reasonable prognosis and reliably predict reasonable development in the children I worked with at the facility.

Here are a few examples to provide clarity and questions for further inquiry.

As you know, I worked with children suffering from traumatic brain injuries, yet each presented different neurological issues. One child was recovering from a coma after a car accident and experienced neural storming. A second experienced ischemic anoxia after hiding in a closet during an apartment fire. The third had tearing and shearing caused by abuse from an angry and frustrated parent. All three children had brain injuries, but each experienced very different types of neural damage. I also served several children with birth defects, including a partial cerebral cortex, a missing hippocampus, and one surviving with just a brain stem. Additionally, I treated a variety of children with generalized pervasive developmental disorders including autism spectrum diagnosis and seizure disorders. As seen through the lens of the Transformational Design Model, this diverse set of children with their differing diagnoses share neurological disorders in common.

I would like to introduce the issues of diagnosis, diagnostic implications, assessment options and paradigm, and treatment approaches through the lives of three children. I will then describe this model's relevance to the adult population. Only then can clinicians begin to put together an appropriate and effective treatment regimen. In this process, I will examine the needs and treatment recommendations for each patient as well as examine the programs that local, state, and federal bureaucracies set up to "support" these children. It is my hope to provide clarity and recommendations to more efficiently and effectively rehabilitate clients in our care. Finally, I will describe a proposed model to financially empower the individuals, their guardians, or representative payees, whatever the financial set up may be.

Chapter One

Dan

Dan is now almost five years old, but when we first met, he was only two. He did not walk or crawl, spoke nothing but the word "Elmo," and screamed and hit his head when anyone interacted with him. Why is this? The first thing that comes to mind for most people is that Dan is displaying a purely behavioral issue caused by environmental triggers and sustained by reinforcements. Cognitively, from this perspective, Dan does not wish to communicate or interact, and he cannot control his responses due to a lack of understanding.

The special education professional responsible for his Individual Education Plan (IEP) assesses the child using best practices prescribed by institutions of public education. The findings label Dan as severely developmentally disabled. Dan is unable to identify colors, numbers, or letters. In addition, he is unable to use language to verbalize familiar objects or to request preferred items. There are additional concerns because of his motor delay, as he cannot crawl, walk, or consistently use his arms in functional motor control. Poor motor skills require him to be tube fed.

The natural conclusion from the traditional perspective

is to begin a regimen of task analysis wherein the teacher breaks down the elements of the skill and uses repetition and reinforcement to practice each element. With this method, Dan experiences occasional success. Success and failure are intermingled with screaming and head slapping. Dan never repeats the appropriate element or skill more than 50 percent of the time, and usually, his success rate is much less than 50 percent. Yet the professionals are satisfied with this progress, and lack of success is attributed to his "stubbornness."

From a behavioral perspective, changing behavior requires the teacher to extinguish the inappropriate behaviors prior to continuing further training, and then, when the negative behaviors are extinguished or eliminated, the teacher reinforces new appropriate behaviors. The teacher may use time outs to remove Dan from the immediate environment, in order to not reinforce the unwanted behavior. As undesired behaviors represent a barrier to learning, this process must be controlled and continuous over a long and repetitive period of time.

Dan must also receive traditional physical and speech therapy. These therapists address motor movement, eating, and language delays. While these motor and language skills are vital in the early development of most children, many of these professional therapists are not trained in neural-sensory processing. As a result, the general conclusion from these therapists is that Dan is not ready or really cannot make significant enough gains to warrant the doctor's prior authorization for Medicaid reimbursement for their clinical services.

A neuroscience perspective provides better diagnostics and treatments that are more effective in helping Dan.

From a neurological standpoint, Dan was born without a hippocampus, which means he cannot transfer recent experiences processed in his short-term or working memory to long-term memory. It also means he cannot coordinate motor movements, resulting in his inability to crawl, walk, or produce verbal responses. Though Dan is able to recognize sounds, he is unable to remember the meaning of these sounds required to create language and communicate. From this neurologic perspective, Dan's screaming and head-slapping are not behavioral issues but responses to the frustration he experiences from being constantly bombarded with inconsistent and constantly novel information (as nothing can be transferred to long-term memory to become permanently learned).

Every time a therapist works with Dan to improve on the 50 percent accuracy gains he acquired in previous sessions, Dan screams and slaps his head. Without a hippocampus, Dan is unable to recall ever learning the skills, movements, or concepts acquired in each previous training session. It is almost as though he never learned anything before. From the traditional therapist's point of view, any gain for Dan is considered a success, but in truth, Dan only approaches success 50 percent of the time (and as noted, usually less than that). At the very best, Dan's rate of success illustrates chance.

A clinician enters. In this case, the clinician is me, armed with Neurologic Music Therapy (NMT) knowledge and the Transformational Design Model. The clinician sees the picture differently and applies standardized and researched diagnostic differentiation assessments and interventions. The first task is to assess Dan from the perspective of hippocampus functions. Since Dan's hippocampus does not exist, the NMT clinician designed the functional skills or movement patterns that traditionally targeted the brain regions responsible for motor control. For the NMT, rhythm (auditory or perceptual) initiates movement.

Physical movement serves to activate neurons in different and specialized parts of the spinal cord. Activated neurons in the spinal cord engage neurons in the brain, including regions dedicated to speech. These regions include both the motor aspects of speech (moving the mouth and tongue) and context elements of speech (semantics or word meaning and syntax, which means word order). Dan's physical movements in response to various rhythms became coordinated, organized, and predictable, providing evidence that he perceived, processed, and remembered the sequences.

The first stage of intervention was to use music to facilitate movement, and the movement produced targeted spinal and then brain or cortical arousal. Music is first perceived through the auditory tract and at the sensory, subcortical level of the brain stem.

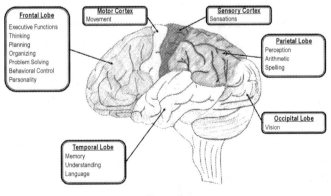

Figure A

A consistent pattern of rhythm is processed in the central nucleus of the amygdala and sent out to the entire brain. I introduced a specific motor pattern, which was immediately followed by Dan rocking forward and back to the wordless tune of "Row, Row, Row Your Boat." Simultaneously in the same session, Dan was introduced and further cortically aroused with a simple tune identifying body parts as they were identified in song lyrics and gently squeezed. I squeezed his shoulders first, then elbows, and then hands. I continued, bilaterally squeezing his hips, knees, and then feet. Second, I introduced a simple marching tune along with a squeeze to alternating feet.

Continuing in succession, Dan was encouraged to stand to a simple ascending scale. According to Thaut (2005) at the Center for Biomedical Research in Music at the University of Toronto, rhythm facilitates timing of movement. The timing and changing intensity of the music is intrinsically connected to coordination of movement and motor patterns. Finally, the term *entrainment* describes a process in which the neural motor system automatically adjusts motor neurons to match the auditory rhythm. This phenomenon has become a standard in Parkinson's gait training across America and has been adopted by the World Federation of Neural Rehabilitation (WFNR) as a clinical standard of practice.

The following is a sample of what a treatment plan may include for a diagnosis like Dan's.

Long-term goals:
1. Dan will produce patterns of motor activity to rhythmic auditory stimuli (RAS).
2. Dan will vocalize along with musical exercises.

3. Dan will complete sessions with absence of body slapping and screaming.

Short-term goals:
1. Dan will tolerate body identification song and motor priming each session with absence of body slapping and screaming.
2. Dan will initiate three specific movements with specific auditory music cues: rocking forward and back, bilateral marching, and sit to stand.
3. Dan will vocalize along with one song per session.

Using Rhythmic Auditory Stimuli (RAS), Music Sensory Orientation (MSOT), and Patterned Sensory Enhancement (PSE) (Thaut, 2005), the NMT's initial step is to assess the child for response to the music and rhythm. As I identified the correct rhythm, Dan re-engaged with me, and within three weeks, he completed twenty to thirty minutes of therapy. Dan vocalized on pitch, recalling and singing the now familiar tunes, clapping hands and knees in perfect rhythm and marching in time while seated. With a change to the musical stimuli and the rhythm, Dan rocked forward and back to the tune of "Row, Row, Row Your Boat." When I stopped the tune and hummed an ascending scale, Dan stood up and cheered on the first time and without prompting. Finally, the NMT combines all three actions into one composition, and when I did this, Dan instantly completed the entire pattern of three movements without prompting or cuing to change the movements.

With the correct application of music and rhythmic stimuli to a properly assessed and diagnosed neurological problem, change occurs quickly and not over months or even years. After four weeks, Dan demonstrated success in gross motor function and for motor function for speech and eating. Dan was able to walk and run freely. He maintained attention in his special classroom, speaking almost anything he needed to, and could eat independently by mouth rather than by G-tube.

The power of PSE and MSOT facilitated proper brain arousal, sustained attention, and provided a catalyst for neural plasticity, completely bypassing his missing hippocampus. This approach served to enhance neural connectivity, which produced remarkable results for Dan in a much shorter time than Applied Behavior Analysis and without the exhausting repetition required by the traditionalist's approach.

Andrew

Andrew is a fifteen-year-old young man who came to the day facility school setting nine months ago. He had just completed a seven-month inpatient stay in intensive care at a children's hospital. Andrew was a typically developing boy who had been cut down by a car while goofing around with his buddies near the road. The discharge report from the hospital diagnosed him with a score of three on the Glasgow Coma scale, otherwise known as a vegetative state. Andrew also had neural storming, which meant his neurons fired constantly and chaotically. This diagnosis resulted in little or no chance of any real recovery, as Andrew did not exhibit any observable behavioral response to environmental stimuli.

How is it possible to assess internal responsiveness

without outward behavioral actions? Does lack of motor or verbal responses provide evidence that Andrew would never interact with his environment because of this injury?

A brief review of literature explains that in some cases, lack of movement reflects a lack of brain activity. Without the use of a Functional Magnetic Resonance Imaging machine (FMRI), which measures brain activity by detecting changes associated with blood flow, it is difficult to measure the degree to which the brain is fully aware despite the body's inability to reflect that awareness. Voss et al., (2006) and Owen and Coleman (2008) shed a little more light on arousal and awareness studies of the injured brain. In their research, they explain that some people in a vegetative state are indeed conscious and aware but unable to physically respond or reflect their consciousness, which is a phenomenon called Locked in Syndrome (Kubler et al., 2009; Kubler & Kotchoubey, 2007; Kubler & Neumann, 2005).

Locked in Syndrome describes those who experience full consciousness and awareness, yet are unable to move or speak in such a way as to communicate their conscious existence to others. In other words, these individuals are unable to communicate their wants, needs, or desires to those they depend on for their very survival. At worst, those with Locked in Syndrome simply exist and because their behavior or language is absent, they cannot receive the treatment reflecting their inherent and conscious dignity. Music sensory orientation training (MSOT) (Thaut, 2005; Magee, 2007; Petacchi, Fox, & Bower, 2005; Graham, 2004; Noda, Maeda, &Yoshino,2004; Sacks, 1998; & Purdie, 1997) has demonstrated the ability to facilitate awake and conscious states among those most severely impaired or injured.

How does Andrew's case differ from that of Dan's case illustrating a missing hippocampus?

Andrew's case did not require initiating movement to achieve neural plasticity. Instead, for Andrew it was necessary to engage functional brain modules (cortical and subcortical) in an organized presentation, to initiate his measurable physical responses to the rhythm. In neuroscience lingo, it was necessary to use external stimuli (rhythm) to effect perception. Addressing perception allowed me to use rhythm to facilitate initiation of, and to sustain Andrew's attention (Thaut, 2005).

How do we know if the patient can perceive the rhythm or whether he hears it?

The neuroscience concept of motor priming involves rhythmically squeezing the individual's joints, which in turn serves to activate motor neurons that jump-start physical movement. Physical movement can be trained to be exhibited in specifically timed and sequenced patterns (Jeong et al., 2007; Dozza et al., 2006; Dozza et al., 2005; McCombe & Whitall, 2005; Luft et al., 2004; Thaut et al., 2002; Yasuhara et al., 2001; Whitall et al., 2000; Effenberg & Mechling, 1998; Paccetti et al., 1998). In Andrew's case, motor priming activated the motor neurons, which engaged his perception. Over the course of three weeks, three times a day for only 15 minutes each time, I sang to Andrew gently squeezing his shoulders, elbows, and hands bilaterally in time with a metronome. Second, I squeezed the hips, knees and feet in the same order while singing, "You can feel your body," and identifying each body part as

I squeezed, first squeezing both sides at the same time and then crisscrossing from right shoulder and left foot, etc.

During the first two weeks, Andrew began to vocalize, which the other therapy staff interpreted as random responses or the expression of discomfort and pain. On the Wednesday of the third week, after completing the priming protocol, Andrew turned his head to meet mine and asked, "How are you?" Since that time, eight months ago, he progressed to singing familiar tunes that he knew prior to the accident, he held conversations about teenaged topics, flirted with the nurses, and sang all the tunes that were played while he was "in a coma."

He demonstrated a plethora of smaller accomplishments including improved flexibility, voluntary motor control, increased strength and endurance and reduced fatigue. He independently exhibited full range of motion and rotation with his right arm and, prompted by a couple of squeezes to his left shoulder, he displayed nearly full range of motion. After rhythmic squeezing, his clenched left fist began to open and close independently in rhythm to the music. His limited, slurred speech only used when cued developed into self-initiated, conversational, and occasionally incessant with affective intention, including a smile. Each week Andrew shared a new trick or song with a new friend in his school. In Andrew's case, rhythmic auditory stimuli (RAS) proved powerful in activating the structures that facilitated initiation, sustained movement, and inhibition of the required neural sequences. Andrew's brain needed consistent sensory input at the subcortical level to engage the Ascending Reticular Activating System (ARAS) as well as the Ascending Reticular Inhibitory System (ARIS), both of which are responsible for starting and stopping neural sequences. In Andrew's case, initiating and inhibiting these neural sequences resulted in his ability to move. Rhythm was the key external stimuli necessary to facilitate the initiation of neural sequences necessary to build levels of attention known as consciousness and communication.

See Figure B.

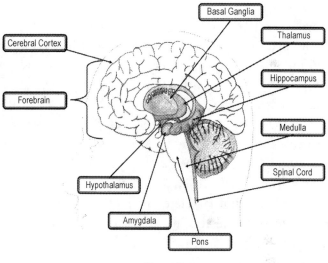

Figure B

Taking a short journey into Andrew's brain, imagine for a moment being a musical creation consisting of only rhythm and melody undergirded with a strong metronome beat. The first step is to enter Andrew's ear canal, where you meet the first roadblock. You are going to bounce a bit as music smacks the tympanic membrane and hesitates because of this barrier. Fortunately, the musical presence and energy continues to activate the eardrum, creating a sound wave through the ossicle bones and oval window and into Andrew's cochlea. Inside this snail-shaped organ, music engages hair-like nerves appropriate for the musical energy level and becomes transformed into electrical impulses. Interestingly, musical energy does not go directly to the brain. Instead, it takes a special side journey to the kidneys to reduce the stress hormone cortisol. Music energy then travels back to the brain stem to jump-start the amygdala located in the anterior temporal lobe. The amygdala connects to many brain regions, including (but not limited to) the thalamus, hypothalamus, hippocampus, and brain stem. These connections allow Andrew to get his groove on, regulating nerve impulses to interpret and match the musical rhythm. This is what I call the "doing the arousal and orientation dance" and two brain structures play an important role: the Ascending Reticular Activation System (ARAS) and the Ascending Reticular Inhibitory System (ARIS). These systems are located in the mid-brain and facilitate initiation and inhibition of responses. They are also instrumental in communicating with other necessary regions of the brain responsible for specific functions.

With this, Andrew has awareness and movement. Andrew will use his previous experience, knowledge and internal control processes to choose how to respond to the music and the multitude of other environmental experiences demanding his attention. Andrew's newly awakened attention now allows him to decide what to attend to, what not to attend to and what to keep an eye on for future response. Presuming of course, Andrew has previous learning and experiences.

Following is the sample treatment plan for Andrew:

Long-Term Goals:
1. Andrew will exhibit sustained attention control.
2. Andrew will produce consistent motor responses to environmental stimuli.

Short-Term Goals:
1. Andrew will orient his body, head or limbs to auditory stimuli twice per session.
2. Andrew will vocalize on rhythmic auditory cues.
3. Andrew will exhibit movement after rhythmic motor priming.
4. Andrew will initiate movements from familiar musical stimuli.

What is the purpose for this set of long- and short-term goals?

In brief, given Andrew's diagnosis of compromised perception and initiation, the goals required external stimuli to reorient his brain and to reconnect and initiate a given quantity of responses. This exercise and method is called Music Sensory Orientation Training (MSOT) and focuses on the quantity of responses required to guide Andrew toward vigilance or awareness over time. Once vigilance was achieved, the therapeutic plan shifted to specifically target levels of attention and increased quality of responses. This particular technique is called Music Attention Control Training (MACT). Once reaching Andrew's optimal level, which in this case took a couple of months of short daily interventions, the therapeutic focus shifted to self-initiation of vocal and motor responses and self-engaging in the classroom activities. There are three specific areas of focus in this stage of therapy:

1. Sustained Attention
2. Divided Attention
3. Alternating Attention

The following is a sample of the second set of long- and short-term goals:

Long-term goals:
1. Andrew will clearly communicate his needs and thoughts.
2. Andrew will use motor control to complete functional motor tasks.
3. Andrew will sustain consistent awareness, orientation and vigilance to the environment.

Short-term goals:
1. Andrew will complete song phrases initiated by external rhythmic stimuli.
2. Andrew will complete 15 minutes of successive vocal tasks to complete classroom performance.
3. Andrew will initiate both upper extremities (BUE) motor tasks on rhythm between two targets with increased speed and accuracy.
4. Andrew will sustain motor tasks for 15 minutes during classroom activities.

This phase of Andrew's treatment took a few months as well, but because of the staff and environmental demands, he only received three 15-minute sessions per day. A more intensive and targeted regimen would have certainly shortened his recovery time and accelerated his progress.

After completing this second set of long- and short-term

goals, Andrew made quick gains in self-initiated verbal conversation, singing, and participation in all classroom activities. In addition, he developed great peer relationships with the other children that originally only gathered around his nearly lifeless body during the initial recovery. Andrew recalled their names, recognized them by their voices and even indicated that some of these peers were closer friends than others. He began letting his original personality shine through and often shared a healthy dose of sassiness. One example was his request to wrestle me while I lay on the floor near him encouraging him to reach, explore his surroundings, and use his ears to identify musical targets. He even got in a little trouble from a few nurses for being a little fresh with his hands during his medical treatments.

Interestingly, Andrew's flirtations serve to undermine the traditional behavioral assumptions. Punishment serves to oppress or limit an overt responsive behavior to a stimulus, therefore reducing the likelihood that a movement will continue. For Andrew, movement was essential for consciousness and inhibiting his activity would, in turn, reduce his consciousness. Neurologic Music Therapy (NMT) offers a better scientific approach to more quickly rehabilitate an injured client requiring overt action to initiate consciousness. I encourage the traditional therapist to consider whether a learned behavior or a neurologic motor response is required for a healing unconscious brain. A quantity of responses is necessary to foster and accelerate progress. Delving into this concept a bit deeper, if quantity of responsiveness is of first importance, punishment or firm disapproval, yelling or scolding, inhibits that progress or stops it in its place.

Eric

Eric is now a 10-year-old boy. A little more than three years ago we met. He also joined the program after an extensive hospital stay. Firefighters had found Eric in a closet after they extinguished a fire in his apartment. Brain scans corroborated the medical team's belief that Eric lacked cortical brain activity. He failed to exhibit any reflexives, including plantar or knee jerk; nor did he exhibit responses to noxious stimuli. Eric was confined to a wheelchair or lying on the floor. Because Eric was unable to display any type of response, I was again confronted with the problem of using an assessment that relies solely on age appropriate behavioral responses.

A review of literature on the assessment of unresponsive individuals failed to provide any definitive answers (Zasler, 1999). A team of NMT practitioners joined together in an effort to use external auditory and tactile stimuli to provide patterns of sensory stimulation. I hypothesized that through this auditory and tactile hierarchy of stimuli Eric would regain or recover some level of orientation and he would demonstrate consistent responsiveness to his environment. Recall Dan, who initially responded to the world with screaming and head slapping and Andrew who responded by moving and moaning. Both these boys initially responded to external stimuli. Eric, however, didn't even reflexively respond to his environment. In all three cases, the therapist initially used the same techniques including patterns of auditory stimuli paired with singing and squeezing joints. NMT worked for Eric because, despite his lack of reflexes and brain activity, his spinal cord and brain were still intact. Recall being music in

Andrew's brain for a moment. Once auditory nerves cells in the inner ear were activated, music energy continued throughout the entire central nervous system. Auditory perception of rhythm imbedded in music fundamentally drives brain function and herein lies the intrinsic power of music perception on human brain function. In Eric's case, the NMT team could identify how and when particular music stimuli and/or music action would engage and change Eric's neural functioning.

Eric progressed slowly, first eating by mouth, then attending a special school simulating regular classroom activity, and self-sitting in the (W) position. He made relatively quick gains over one year, but then seemed to hit a plateau, which I did not accept as the end of his progress.

Could the traditional classroom help or potentially harm Eric's recovery?

Consider for a moment the possibility that when facilitating recovery or reorganization of an erased brain, a regular classroom environment, structured to support the neural typical brain, would be harmful to Eric's development. A regimen of applied behavioral analysis methods, designed to gain a consistent response to a single stimulus, engraves a parietal frontal loop between limbic emotions and subcortical sensory processing, bypassing the rest of the thinking brain. Eric did not learn to think, plan, or organize, but instead responded reflexively to conditioned stimuli. After the trauma, Eric's cognitive brain was erased, functioning much like that of a newborn. He had no possibility of recovering previously learned movement, sustained attention, thinking, memory or communication. Though his brain was searching for patterns of stimuli to attend to, many of those patterns were overwhelming, causing his awareness to shut down or sleep. Eric was bombarded with hyper-sensory stimulation similar to a parent reading Dickens to a newborn. His teachers repeated colors and letters, numbers and shapes to his newborn intellect, reinforcing his responses with candy. Considering Eric's lack of response in light of the other cases discussed, use of new assessments, understanding and clinical application to each individual's needs should guide planning, programming, and structures of support to promote growth.

Let us consider this neurologic explanation of functioning and then an appropriate neural-sequential approach to recovery.

Sample Treatment Plan

Long-term Goals:
1. Eric will attend to and interact with his environment with patterned responses and interaction.

Short-term Goals (60 days):
1. Eric will self-engage in MSOT (music sensory orientation training, (Level 2 orientation) consistently for 15-minute session each day exhibited by head orientation to visual, tactile and auditory rhythmic stimulation.
2. Eric will consistently respond to MSOT (Music Sensory Orientation Training, (Level 1 arousal) responding to rhythmic auditory stimulation for 15 minute session each day.
3. Eric will exhibit bilateral balance from hip support through Rhythmic Auditory Stimuli (RAS) and

Therapeutic Instrumental Music Performance (TIMP) exhibited by sitted self-support and upper trunk control.

Short-Term Goals (120 days):
1. Eric will maintain head control for 10 minutes per class activity each day exhibited by eye contact at task or staff.
2. Eric will improve Both Upper Extremities (BUE) control exhibited by hitting target strikes 50 percent of trials.
3. Eric will sit up from forward lying independently 50 percent of trials.

Short Term Goals (90 days):
1. Eric will maintain head control, directed at session task and staff for 90 percent of each NMT session.
2. Eric will direct Both Upper Extremities (BUE) to session tools upon request and with musical stimuli 75 percent of trials.
3. Eric will sit up independently 100 percent of trials with request or tactile cue.

After implementing these goals Eric began making new gains in recovery, including faster responses to patterned auditory stimuli. He also vocalized and followed ascending or descending vocal patterns and moved his upper body in rhythm with the music. His movements became organized, targeted and controlled.

In the case of Eric, who had no responses, the goal was to increase the quantity of responses rather than the quality of responses. This stands in complete opposition to the theories and philosophies held by traditional therapists and special educators. According to the research of Thaut (2015) in the recovery of wake states or original development of wake states or sustained attention, it is vital to use appropriately selected patterns of stimuli. In addition, because we could not ascertain if there was even perception of our interaction, it was also vital to use motor priming and tactile interventions to drive central nervous system functions. Like an infant, Eric was reborn. He needed to begin the process of brain development through the same approaches used with infants and toddlers. Consider again how the traditional team would approach treatment using cultural norms rather than neurologic principles.

A common buzz phrase is, "Everything must be age appropriate." The question should be, "Chronological age or functional age?"

Additionally, Eric was taught in a setting that included full inclusion. Full inclusion is intended to give those with special needs more opportunity and resources by including them with their non-disabled peers. This one-size-fits-all, blanket approach to education does not meet the individualized neurological needs of children with special needs like those discussed in this book. In a later chapter, I'll discuss in detail the myths, conflicts and potential damage caused by the past special education, Individualized Education Plan, No Child Left Behind, and Common Core decisions or approaches.

Again, I'll ask the question: would you enroll your infant or toddler in a classroom designed for six-, seven-, or eight-year-old—or older—children?

The simple answer is that you would not; an infant's brain is not ready for that level of stimuli.

Now for a moment, let's contrast Eric's approach with that of Andrew's. Andrew initially needed some quantity of stimuli for arousal to bring him out of the unorganized neural storming after the concussive brain injury. He then quickly shifted to improving and increasing quality of responses including motor, cognition, recall, and increasing vigilance, and fostering self-initiation of response to environment.

Eric is now actively self-engaging with the classroom environment exhibited by several key responses. First, when he hears me enter the room in my typical loud arrival he begins squealing with happiness. In addition, if he is not strapped into his wheelchair, he begins bouncing excitedly. A second example of him becoming personally engaged blooms when a group or other therapy is occurring nearby. Again, if he isn't strapped in and immobilized, when he hears me working with others he hightails it over to our area by either rolling, somersaulting, or using a rapid bounce and scoot maneuver. He'll then immediately sit up in W-sitting and vocalize/sing and bounce along with the music.

Nick

I first met Nick when he was one year old after recently being discharged from the neonatal intensive care unit (NICU) at a children's hospital. Shortly after his birth he was rushed to the children's hospital, unresponsive. His diagnosis was a severe and unusual seizure disorder and scans showed almost constant seizure activity. He had no observable response to the environment. The monitor in his crib displayed a very low heart rate, oxygen levels were at or below 80 percent and staff could not visually see the rise and fall of his chest. As a result, his lungs filled with fluid quickly and the nurses hovered waiting to provide the suction necessary to keep him from aspirating. During the first few weeks at the medical childcare facility, he was frequently readmitted to the NICU with chronic pneumonia and respiratory infections.

I began NMT planning to assist with facilitating wakefulness and arousal states. I hoped that improved arousal and orientation would decrease seizure activity. Previous music therapy research revealed inconsistent heart and respiration rate responses to music (Music for stress and anxiety reduction in coronary heart disease patients, Bradt & Dileo, 2009 & 2013). Again, I implemented the motor priming approach of Music Sensory Orientation Training (MSOT) in theory to foster consistent quantity of responsiveness. I sang wordless melodies with the metronome while squeezing his joints; a pattern similar to that used with the other clients. This immediately brought his respiration and heart rate as well as oxygenation levels to normal ranges. That meant he had oxygen saturation levels near or at 100 percent and significant increases in heart rate. Staff could visually watch the rise and fall of his chest as he breathed deeper during NMT interventions. Whenever his stats fell, the nurses called my cell phone and over I rushed to intervene and each time his vital signs returned to normal levels. After a few weeks Nick consistently attended the medical childcare program.

Is this a permanent change in Nick's health? Is Nick just making temporary progress during the intervention? Can Nick's vital signs be maintained with creating a controlled sensory environment?

Whenever he returned to the medical daycare program, I implemented the NMT protocol and his stats normalized. Very quickly his stats held near normal and the number of invasive medical suction or even deep suction decreased in frequency. A couple of months prior to his second birthday, Nick began to vocalize along with the melodies he and I enjoyed together during that first year. The nursing staff gathered around with smiles and shock. His previously tense little body, with both arms and legs stiff as a board in seizure activity, began to relax along with descending patterns of song. Rhythmic Auditory Stimuli (RAS) began to cue and change specific motor responses to the music. His little arms would rise with the first line of "Twinkle, Twinkle, Little Star," and lower to a relaxed position with the second phrase. Nick quickly advanced from singing the last note of each phrase to completing the entire scale. He also developed increased motor control to include patterned flexion and extension of both arms. The metronome marked time in the background while I tapped his elbows. As I sang a verse of "Row, Row, Row Your Boat" he bent both elbows in time with the music and touched hands together at his belly midline. As I continued the verse, he independently extended both arms. Change the song, and he squeezed and released his little fingers around my own. The nursing staff could finally relax and spend more time with the other children in the unit.

Chapter Two

Historical Child Development and Education Model

For most of America's history, school systems and settings were exclusive rather than today's approach of inclusion. Initially educational exclusion was due to several factors including ignorance, prejudice and even racism rooted in fear. Yet now inclusive education reflects a lack of intellectual vigor. Inclusion can and will ill-serve the education systems, particularly if it is yoked with the powerful unions' blind ideology.

Everyone is familiar with the story of Laura Ingalls' schoolhouse, which describes children studying near a warm cozy fire at home or at the little red schoolhouse located in the country on a hill in or near the edge of town. In this version of education, children scurry in from miles around to master their lessons from patient teachers trained in standard pedagogy. The truth is these stories exclude the forgotten ones: children of all ages with disabilities who were either kept home out of embarrassment or removed from sight and mind and moved to institutions or worse, eliminated. Establishment of civil liberties in the middle 20th century changed exclusion for some, but not all, students. The groundbreaking events and legal battles included Brown versus Board of Education, U.S. (1954). The United States Supreme Court case declared that state laws establishing separate public schools for black and white students were unconstitutional - a ruling overturning an almost 100-year older decision, Plessy v. Ferguson of 1896, which allowed state-sponsored segregation in public education. However, in May of 1954, the Warren Court ruled unanimously that separate educational settings were unconstitutional. This action proved a major step forward in the civil rights movement to eliminate legalized racial segregation. Integration and inclusion were on the move in education for this changing society.

While this early movement was a pivotal development in American history, it was limited in scope and only began a change in education for African Americans. An often-forgotten minority group had to wait for almost two decades for a similar movement. The disabilities community did not receive legal recognition and opportunity until the Individualized Education Plan (IEP) process of 1975 during the Nixon and Ford administration. The IEP process is and was designed to focus on the needs of the individual child, as opposed to protecting a relatively anonymous group of African American children. Despite individual differences, the disabled students were required to be included in gathering outcome data through standardized assessments and testing. Once more, according to the new law, the IEP closely aligned with the regular education curriculum.

Out of this trend, mainstreaming began in the 1980's during the Reagan administration. Even then, mainstreaming was reserved for the least disabled children. Most severely disabled children and adults were removed from their families and institutionalized or separated from their typically developing peers. Special education classrooms and resource rooms began to spring up to teach and train skills specific to the individual student's needs. The blind or visually impaired (as in my case) learned skills like mobility, Braille and typing in one classroom and then joined the typically developing students in math, science or physical education classes. Often accompanied by a support staff, the disabled children sat quietly in the back of a classroom listening (or oftentimes not listening) to the regular education curriculum. The disabled students then returned to their resource room to complete lessons in modified academics to keep them close in achievement to their non-disabled peers. Again, this was only for the few that were thought to be ready for such a transition.

Let's spend a few minutes discussing the IEP, the foundation of any model of special education today.

What is it, and what are the key elements of the "individualized" plan?

First, the IEP is designed to be individualized, specific for the student. IEPs are to ensure that every child with a disability has access to the same educational opportunities as their non-disabled peers. School districts then will provide and support any necessary modifications and adaptations to assist with student success. The interdisciplinary team is to set goals together that will guide the education program for the year. That plan will be implemented according to the needs of each child and reviewed by professionals that are also identified in that plan. Each student's team may be comprised of different experts based upon the needs and request of the individual student and his or her family. Together the team creates a plan which becomes an official document or contract outlining the rehabilitation, support, academic adaptations or other resources required to achieve the student's individualized goals. The plan is funded by the school district.

Key elements must be identified here and emphasized:

1. The plan must be individualized for the needs of the student;
2. The goals and outcomes must include the input and direction of the student and his or her family;
3. The team must be defined based upon the needs and wishes of the student and family;
4. The team is responsible for ensuring the student and family have every opportunity to be successful;
5. Any team member, including the family, can reconvene and make requests to adjust the plan at any time; and
6. The school district is responsible for the cost of educating and providing financial payment for everything delineated in the IEP.

Notice several common elements in the previous list of key elements. The repeated theme is "the student and the family." The law empowers students and their families to drive the IEP and outcomes, not just the professionals that represent the school, therapists, medical personnel or the rest of the members of the team. The school and team members' responsibilities should center on the student and they are there to provide their "expertise" by helping provide an individualized curriculum and to make sure it happens in a reasonable and appropriate way. Those responsibilities include funding those needs and not simply replicating a plan used for other students in the same age range or shared disability.

In 1997, The Individuals with Disabilities Education Act (IDEA) was passed to provide "strengthening to the earlier laws and procedures." The premise of this act was based upon the theory that all children can learn and grow within the current education system and would be successful with support. Support in this case means additional accommodations and the funding required to finance support.

These educational supports and approaches were based upon behavioral explanations of learning. For example, a middle school teacher of mine used to begin our English class by asking each day: "What is the key to instruction?" The class then responded each day "repetition, upon repetition, with even more repetition." This was a very powerful approach for concept development for the traditional student, with a traditionally working brain or central nervous system (CNS). The children with special needs were presumed to require more repetition to learn or grasp concepts. Education used Skinnerian methods to achieve results. Applied Behavioral Analysis (ABA) utilizing a stimulus response approach presents the stimuli and then repeats the stimuli until the appropriate response to stimuli appears and then immediately reinforces that response.

This is very effective way to teach a rat to push a lever to get a food reward. The only problem is that children, with or without disabilities, are not rats. Nor do they have brains that are the same as rats'. In most cases the human brain has additional features, complexities and abilities. I state, "in most cases" because there are instances where brain dysfunction is due to missing brain regions. Such was the case with the example of Dan without short-term memory. In his case, ABA or any repetitive model could not work and a different approach was necessary.

The standard educational model also presumes that age is an indicator of readiness to learn particular skills or concepts. A common phrase used in the industry is "age appropriate" - for example, in kindergarten the five-year-old learns "A B C" while the first grade child learns $1 + 2 = 3$. Age, however, can be defined both chronologically and developmentally. Readiness for skills and concepts should be based on diagnostics as opposed to age.

Another development and trend that has swept up the disabilities community is the "Lovaas" method (Lovaas, 1987; McEachin, Smith, & Lovaas, 1993). This method brought in new excitement and changed approaches for the growing epidemic of autism now more commonly known as Autism Spectrum Disorders or ASD. The Lovaas method is a standardized pattern of ABA theory; again, somewhat effective to gain a specific response to a specific stimulus after lots of consistent and structured experience and training. An unfortunate result has been a significant growth in obsessive "behaviors" ensconced in brains trained like the rats. Recent neural science research has shown that this method does little more than engrain brain loops from sensory awareness areas of the brain to emotional centers and back and forth. A recent article on optimizing brain functioning by identifying and addressing presence of primitive reflexes that failed to inhibit after birth, reveals fundamental needs in brain development. It also highlights a need for change in the system to properly identify and address these issues (Balasubramani, & Hayden, 2018).

The concept of back and forth is important to understand because this neural sequence appears as a repetitive and obsessive behavior. That's right, we caused the obsessive compulsive behavior and then need to develop another approach to extinguish the new undesirable behavior.

Another way to describe it may be that we've just taught the rat to push the lever and now he can't stop pushing the lever! A well-known autism advocate, Dr. Temple Grandin (1992) has described the awful result of the autism experience as she describes her personal squeeze box. She designed this piece of equipment to regain her personal sense of self. When the brain is trapped in the neurologic loop of emotions, memories and sensory perception, the individual often loses complete awareness of the rest of the body. Dr. Suzanne Oliver, NMT Fellow, states how this often results in body slapping, hitting, stomping of feet or throwing oneself on the floor. These actions are not a negative behavior as most commonly assessed, but the individual's attempt to regain awareness of the body's extremities.

What this has fostered is a broken system of special education, attempting to force underdeveloped or damaged brains to produce results we haven't enabled them to experience, because of our adherence to tradition, not science and truth.

Unfortunately, this pattern of interventions not based on research and data continues today. In 2014 the Obama administration was pushing hard for "Common Core" and Congress was falling in line.

Is this because they don't understand?

Are they doing it on purpose at the expense of the students or to support the powerful unions that cannot afford changes to their golden system?

How can "Common Core" even be considered, much less implemented, given the diagnostic differentiation I've just described?

Each case example described displays the circumstance of so many children across the nation that need accurate assessments and opportunities designed specifically for their brains, nervous systems and functional needs. It is vital to rethink and push back against cookie cutter common core or any new revelation from the system that has consistently failed our children.

So what? ...

The education system has developed an approach that can be very successful in training children or young adults to grow and thrive, if they have the traditional processing brain. Yep, I said processing brain and not the learning brain. Here are a few concepts to consider as we continue, that I will explain in detail after we explore a few more steps in our process and the future of disability services.

1. Three important steps in fostering and supporting growth and development: perception, production and planning.
2. What elements in our world, communities and culture support perception, production and planning?
3. What is it that makes us different from that rat?
4. What in society is it that keeps us from embracing our differences from rats?

The foundational theories for special education include

the Skinnerian theories or applied behavioral analysis, the Lovaas method and traditional approaches like repetition and reinforcement. What this did for the community of children with disabilities is to delay or lose valuable time to enhance independence and skill development, resulting in communities not knowing what to do with all these now grown children with few skills. Large state-run institutions began to develop and fill up across our nation with people with severe disabilities who were mostly warehoused with lots of more applied behavioral treatments. These unfortunate animalized people were trained like rats and therefore acted like rats, unable to differentiate and internalize their individual human existence and purpose. They were able to complete specific tasks under specific environmental controls and never able to generalize and intellectualize the information and experiences.

One example of this approach became evident a decade or so ago when my state began closing the government-run institutions. Most of these wonderful people were diagnosed as profoundly developmentally impaired, yet each of them came to us with a work history and were recommended for vocational evaluations. One individual we met and assessed mostly sat upon a floor in his loose-fitting clothing and Depends. He spent the entire time we observed him flipping a string he had pulled from his clothing up and down. When any of the staff tried to engage him, he screamed and hit his head and stomped his foot. It turns out that his work experience was shifting objects from one box to another. He needed a personal assistant to cue him to initiate the action, however. This was accomplished by slamming a mallet on the table next to the client, which in turn made the consumer scream and move the item from one box to the next. This is defined as work experience. Unfortunately, the professionals trained him to work because "after all, he is of working age" rather than using thoughtfulness, reason and intellect. Traditionalist ideology guides practice rather than research. Also, missing in the equation is the human element, the unique nature of this individual and how creation is structured to form our existence and interaction with it.

Clinicians and staff were — and are still today — unable to include the special human element. We are different creations with very specially designed brains, bodies and purposes. Humans have a limbic system that fills us with detailed memories and emotions including the need to love and be loved. We are also then relational and need human affection aside from animal-driven sexuality.

All of this process doubled down on approaches to drill in responses to stimuli rather than take a closer look at the specific need of the individual brain. I understand that 50, 40, 30 and even 20 years ago we did not have the neural science data research and imaging to identify the flaws in our approaches, but we do now and there is no excuse -- unless the purpose is more related to fundamentally changing our society away from its foundation.

Considering the recent renaissance, let's rethink our traditions and begin to put together a new and more foundationally grounded approach. One-size-fits-all does and should not apply to education, and communities must drive its core, standards and curriculum, not elected leaders from across the state or nation.

The IEP should clearly be individualized and there are several ways this should be done. The family should drive and select the team. Along with the pediatrician, they should address several questions including clarification of the diagnosis, whether the child is able to perceive the environment, and if so; which stimuli and patterns might affect and sustain attention and foster vigilance.

Once the child demonstrates vigilance and attention control is sustained, he or she is able to respond to external stimuli. Additionally, as each phase of development is achieved, the families should reassess which team members are necessary to progress to the next phase of development. This may also mean that some team members may not be beneficial during each level of growth. Somewhat of a radical concept I know, but team membership should be considered to ensure the best use of staff and financial resources.

Another consideration then is how to quantify and measure progress to ensure we are truly accomplishing what we claim to be doing. The current system is using assessments that begin with cognition and a level of executive function; meanwhile, many of our children with disabilities are in another phase known as perception. This phase consists of three specific concepts or functions to be achieved:

1. Arousal: is each individual aware of the surrounding environment through hearing, vision, auditory, kinesthetic and olfactory senses?
2. Orientation: is each individual orienting eyes, head, hands and feet to and at the stimuli?
3. Vigilance: does the individual sustain or maintain attention to each or any of these stimuli?

This initial phase provides some level of difficulty regarding measuring progress, as the only way to assess and measure awareness at this point is through functional imagery. However, if the sensory orientation training is done correctly, using rhythmic auditory and tactile stimuli, observable responses will occur immediately. Movement is among the initial consistent responses to patterned environmental stimuli. Once these responses are present and consistent there are many standardized assessment tools that should be used to quantify results and drive future curriculum and special education planning and goals.

The education establishment believes all children should receive the same resources – regardless of diagnosis "because it's only fair." The traditional educational system must be enlightened and retrained. There needs to be a movement from families and individuals to push the system toward progress and foundational change. This is, of course, somewhat of a paradox. On the one hand, I am advocating for fundamental change and yet, I am returning to older tradition! Still a great "however" remains that I will address as we take a closer look at these developments in light of the diagnosis and needs of our case examples. Then we'll shed some light on the fallacies of blanket policy and egalitarianism, designing "equality" curriculum that flies in the face of IDEA.

It seems to me that equality, the same curriculum, and the same approaches don't belong in every child's plan, since these children may have vastly different perceptual and brain needs.

The following is a general list of standardized assessment tools that can be used to guide and inform treatment and planning beyond initial phases of perception:

1. TRIAD Social Skills Assessment
2. IMTAP Individualized Music Therapy Assessment Profile
3. The Timed Up and Go test (TUG Test)
4. Dynamic Gait Index
5. Functional Reach Test
6. Houser Ambulation Index

Chapter Three

Now we have reached the point where it is clear that system changes are needed and the foundational principles to do so, exist. We can begin to retrain future education leaders in a fuller understanding of the brain. Diagnostic differentiating is vital to individualized training so that each student with his unique nervous system can be supported appropriately. Current approaches are designed to train people to learn and reproduce concepts despite the fact that many children require perceptual training. We can use valid and reliable assessments to identify specific needs for individual children and develop a truly individualized education developmental plan, whatever the need may be.

In contrast, current education programs lack effective and reliable assessment of perception and arousal, orientation and vigilance. Current assessments only focus on academic principles. Additionally, the assessments fail to account for specific brain functions, thwarting the ability to create individualized interventions adapted to meet the needs of each child. This results in plans that fail to take into account the neural sequential steps necessary to achieve rapid and powerful development. Second, the IEP does not include the necessary approaches, team members or financial allocation to foster long-term independence.

Existing models depend on slow and steady progress utilizing intense levels of "supports." The method I have introduced pinpoints need, assigns treatment methods and protocol, achieves immediate results, shifts and modifies treatment based upon predictable outcomes, and decreases time needed for change, thereby reducing cost! This type of specifically structured plan efficiently utilizes the team's skills and resources. Consequently, time, effort and energy can be shifted to other individuals with needs for significantly more point of contact hours.

Following the court actions of the 70's, 80's and 90's, the next trend included closing state-run institutions and moving those individuals to community or residential living. This represented a very positive step for the futures and lives of people with special needs as it afforded people with disabilities greater access to community resources and opportunities. Quick to follow was the intense effort to create community inclusion and integration. Once again, however, it was hoped that people with severe and profound impairments would magically improve through experiences and interaction with non-disabled peers. Bus after bus of unknowing and often unwilling people were loaded up, driven across towns, counties and even states to experience the new frontiers. Unfortunately, as this well-meaning activity was going on, behaviors, outbursts, and indecent exposure began to spoil the fabulous outing.

Why should this happen?

I thought that by common opportunity and financial "supports" that all would be well?

Sound familiar to the last shift in approach?

Everybody will benefit from the multitude of opportunity and experiences.

So, it seems we have now almost completed a full circle of approaches in our early childhood education system. The system has moved from complete isolation, to separate but equal education, to mainstreaming with the Least Restrictive Environment (LRE), to integration and inclusion. What is next?

Let us take another look at our case examples in the scenario of each of these models and what the potential developmental impact would possibly be on each of these people. What would the outcomes possibly be given the special diagnosis of each? What effect would the environment be on each consumer?

Andrew, for example, 30 years ago would have left intensive care after injury in the similar state as he did, however he would not have a specialized school to attend to his medical and educational needs. He also would not have had the benefit of intensive therapies options to support and accelerate his recovery. A state-run institution would most likely have been his first stop, and probably his last. The family and a public school could not have supported his intense medical needs. While living in one of these institutions, he would have had some access to therapies that would have probably set goals appropriate for his functional level, including sensory integration and adaptations to include him in regular groups. There would have undoubtedly been large periods of time where Andrew sat idle and/or alone since he had little to no response. The professionals would have agreed that he may make some slow but steady progress over a long time, but never regain any functional independence.

As the deinstitutionalization movement approached, he may have been moved to a school district with a self-supported special education classroom. Here the staff would have designed a modified curriculum based upon his chronological age and begun teaching concepts with every conceivable adaption. He can't see, so tactile hand over hand concepts may have been used to show him what he was learning. They may have even included sensory integration protocol to introduce various visual, tactile, auditory and olfactory experiences. Given his diagnosis, he may have been able to perceive each of these and even remember what they were, however he probably would have never been able to produce a meaningful response to any of them. He may have also been rolled into English, math and science class to be a part of the regular classroom integrated with his non-disabled peers. Possibly he could have been aware of what occurred and maybe even learned some new concepts, but he certainly would have never been able to show anyone that he had indeed learned anything. He would still be unable to initiate a response to environmental stimuli; meanwhile he also would probably begin slipping further and further into states of unconscious indifference, not having the necessary patterns of environmental stimuli designed for his neurologic needs. He would have needed approaches to effectively initiate and sustain his attention. The least restrictive environment, for him, would have been determined based on the assumption of a neural typical brain. This approach fails to account for the need to regain consistency and speed in arousal, orientation and vigilance. He would have never reached the ability to sustain his own attention and produce meaningful and consistent responses to the world.

A second scenario might have been the Skinnerian approach. Again, this would consist of presenting an antecedent stimulus designed to facilitate a response combined with an immediate reinforcement to increase the likelihood of the response repeating. Andrew indeed had some autonomic responses to stimuli or basic reflexes; however, keep in mind the traditional team concluded he had neural storming and so would not proceed with these interventions until that medical issue was resolved.

Human function in a healthy state implies an integration of motor, emotional, contextual and experiential information. More to the point, human executive function requires a complex coordination of brain regions including perception, motor response, association with previous experience, and then planning and adjustment based upon multiple factors. This entire process may take a fraction of a second. Sensory-based perception can and will occur with complete absence of cognition. In the case of Andrew, he was indeed cognitively aware, but not able to initiate a response. The process of cognition and recognizable evidence of learning and executive functions requires not only the integration of sensory input, its transfer to cortical regions above the subcortex and brain stem, but then also consistent and thoughtful response, coding and decoding of the familiar sensory information, and use and interaction with it. Brain scans of person receiving a positive reinforcement approach show that the sensory input and response area within the subcortex is first engaged; then the limbic system responsible for emotional memory; and then back again to the subcortex; creating a loop that bypasses the rest of the contextual brain necessary for intellectual processing, storage, reason, planning and so on. In a later chapter, I'll discuss the current neuroscience explanation of looping. So, Andrew may have been able to reproduce a specific response to a specific stimuli after reinforcement, but never have been able to generalize it based upon a constantly changing world reality. In addition, his rapid recovery of motor activity and control may have never been developed since that was the means we used to facilitate brain activation and restoration of vital learned skills.

Either approach undoubtedly would have resulted in Andrew sitting in a self-contained classroom, with several staff, educators and therapists trying over and over to gain a consistent response and probably never getting it. Getting responses, certainly, but consistently and improving in quality, never. Once more, because his brain would be looped and limited in global arousal, he would never access the previously learned content that he is now recalling and using every day. These staff would of course say he is making progress, but given his injury it will take a long, long time and they can't say for sure how much he will ever achieve.

Another look forward requires a closer look at the impact of both mainstreaming and inclusion on Andrew.

Given the descriptions of brain function and deficits with initiation and inhibition of cognitive processes, what would he ever reproduce meaningfully from mainstreaming?

If he is in class, possibly learning because he is aware, can the typical special education break out room and its staff facilitate a response that is functional for human interaction?

In an inclusion setting, would he ever communicate his answers to math problems or formulate his understanding of a historical event and what it means for his future decisions and interaction in life?

What would this mean for the system, both the education and long-term support system? What would the projected supports needed for his life expectancy cost, including ongoing rehabilitation, housing, medical, and recreational expenditures? Of course, we may also be considering what costs may be needed to surround him with supports to facilitate work. After the scenario descriptions, we'll take a closer look at estimates of these traditional approaches based upon today's dollars and average costs. We can put real dollar amounts on both the special education and long-term care portions of his expected life span and then calculate a number based upon the alternative model system that is careful to provide diagnostic-based intervention and approaches to brain development. This too would be coupled with targeted staff allocation and assignment, using only professionals with the skill and knowledge to apply research-based approaches with predictable and timely outcomes.

Eric

Once again let us step back several decades and analyze Eric's situation. Right off the bat it is safe to say that had his injury occurred this long ago, he would not have survived the house fire. Thanks to modern advances in every aspect of human life, he did. Second, had he survived he may have been supported in his own family's home, where – hopefully - he would benefit from a supportive and nurturing family environment. This home life may produce slow and steady development given a presumption of the "Leave it to Beaver" setting. As mainstreaming ensued, the setting could have progressed his recovery through interaction, but long periods of academics could not possibly make an impact on him academically and developmentally. Remember, his brain was effectively erased and he needed to begin at the start, with consistent patterns of responsiveness to environmental interaction. Any attempts to educate, using "age appropriate" methods, would have evaded him completely. Like the newborn, the brain needs patterns of arousal, orientation and vigilance. Consequently, each opportunity to mainstream would have been meaningless and ineffective. Likewise, each attempt by a special education professional to adapt curriculum, would also have been ineffective and a waste of Eric's valuable time and society's valuable resources. Furthermore, any time and money spent upon him by the special education teacher would be time and money that could not be spent with another student in the correct stage of development for his or her services. Inclusion then would simply not provide the necessary environment to foster any change to produce the outcomes that would ensure a long-term level of independence and life fulfillment. You see, only very specific and specially trained professionals are equipped to address his needs and by using and maximizing their skills, we also maximize the resources.

Consider this alternative: as Eric is engaged in targeted central nervous system (CNS) interventions, he recognizes staff and daily schedules. As he identifies each one, he responds accordingly, vocalizing pleasure and facilitating mobility to self-engage in these experiences. In this functionally appropriate environment, Eric can be supported to expand and sustain or maintain attention to sensory-based curriculum. As specific motor patterns are developed within the sensory structures, the neural sensitive interventions will accurately engage expanded brain regions. As each of these brain regions are activated, the corresponding observable functional response will occur quickly and consistently. Using the neural sequential approach, through motor priming and sequencing, the team will achieve levels of attention to include sustained, divided, and alternating attention. Consequently, the ever more complex attention and complete cortical arousal will elicit vocal and then verbal responses, especially if the material is sung. Eric then begins to vocalize within a few seconds of musical stimuli in his environment.

In addition, once engaged, he will follow specific ascending and descending patterns and complete musical phrases with the correct note. The significance of phrase completion is his development of the ability to identify, recall, and anticipate the lyric phrase and/or pitch. This neurologic principle of development is known as auditory perception, a higher and more advanced cognitive skill.

Secondly, he is able to shift and modify movement patterns to correspond with specific music stimuli. The four-beat tune of "Row, Row, Row Your Boat," with specific emphasis on alternating "rows," facilitates consistent extension and flexion of the arms, forward and back. Shift the tune to a triple meter, 1, 2, 3, 1, 2, 3, and he immediately begins to rotate the arms in large circles, both out, up, and around, meeting in the middle and then landing on his wheelchair tray. In this therapeutic exercise, there are no verbal directions, just simple sensory auditory cues of force through musical emphasis, rhythmic timing, and sequencing of alternating musical patterns. In this neurological sensory reorganization and interaction, the movement is stimulating motor neurons along the spinal cord and then motor modules in the brain, which in my clinical opinion will begin to expand his communication and verbal ability. "Why?" you may ask. Speech motor modules just so happen to sit adjacent to the motor control centers. By eliciting bilateral motor activity, we realize these immediate vocal responses I referenced earlier. It is all connected and designed that way. An accident? I don't think so.

Dan

Dan's trip through tradition in early intervention methods would be packed with exciting events. Recall, his functional skill levels when therapy was initiated were such that standard clinicians concluded there was little that could be done. His missing hippocampus would simply not allow him to develop the skills necessary to walk or speak. It is somewhat difficult to project what the impact of inclusion and/or mainstreaming would have upon him, as he was just beginning to reach that age of attending regular school. However, one thing is for certain: the traditional system would identify there is little to accomplish because of the diagnosis and the limits of traditional approaches to therapy and education. The default response to the newness of each experience would be head slapping and screaming. Every year of school would be another of less than 50 percent accuracy on goals set during intervention and little progress. Most likely he would always be in a self-contained classroom, but shifted periodically into specially selected inclusive options. These inclusion situations would be exacerbated by the same "negative behavioral" response. The therapy team most likely would conclude the same as ours: we can't make enough progress to warrant a medical prior authorization. You see, neural plasticity is a specialized concept and field of intervention. Even more specialized is a neural sequential plan to address the underlying brain function specific to each diagnosis. The natural approach in today's culture would be a wonderfully designed special classroom full of age appropriate experiences. It would all look good and the community would be pleased with this rosy picture of opportunity. The families would be happy, sort of, about the opportunities; meanwhile internally very frustrated and experiencing the slow pain of realizing their child will never gain functional independence nor the joy of discovery and learning. However disappointing, this is the template and the treatment team's unspoken level of expectation for the child. Families are told, "We'll do everything to offer the experiences to foster long-term development," yet no one ever looks at the consistent effectiveness of the procedure. The student would have developed and achieved more if he was functionally able, they say, rather than asking, "Are the approaches appropriate for the individualized needs?" A few simple examples may help provide clear understanding of the traditional process for Dan. The hippocampus is responsible for transferring learned information from sensory regions and short-term or limbic emotions to cerebral or cognitive/thinking regions where our intellect and executive functions work, thrive, grow, expand and store useful information. So, each classroom learning task was new for him, no matter how many times it was taught. He did not have the sequence of loops to connect the neurons to the higher cognitive brain regions. By using the rhythmic driven motor patterns, we not only elicited immediate motor patterns, but networks reaching the cognitive cortex and thus executive learning. If Dan can hear, recognize and respond with motor patterns to specific musical tunes, he can hear, see and recognize events in the environment and begin to respond appropriately.

Nick

Nick is another example of how the system is unprepared to address his needs. Yes, his needs are vast and difficult, but not unworkable or unworthy of careful and researched planning and implementation. Traditionalists looking at his lifeless body and multiple monitors would conclude, "What can be done?" I have to admit, I thought the same when I first saw him and read his chart. There are two possible responses, I guess. First, try what always was done. Alternatively, take a closer look at the specific diagnosis, what that means in the hierarchy of neurological functioning, and assess for what external stimuli fosters any response. When that specific stimulus is identified, use the knowledge of the human body and nervous system and build those responses little by little and in proper order. This is a child that would probably have never left the hospital and if he did, it would not be to a happy home, but to a processional of tears.

This same child is the one that now sings and moves his

little arms with the music. He eagerly squeezes my fingers according to the sensory intensity of each song. His little elbows and forearms independently flex and extend with each phrase of "Row, Row, Row Your Boat"; meanwhile he smiles and sings. Certainly a vast contrast to the lifeless body of our first meeting!

For now, he still suffers from persistent medical concerns. Because of his inconsistent arousal and orientation, it's as if his little body forgets to breathe deeply and gets a little lazy. However, when he is sensory aroused and engaged, his attention begins and along with that attention, his autonomic system revives. As the vital signs regulate, the oxygen levels normalize, the heart rate slows to normal and his respirations deepen. As the breath deepens, he begins coughing and loosening congestion, coughs it up, and staff can suction as needed and/or Nick can manage the process independently. His lungs clear and hospitalizations reduce as pneumonia is diagnosed less often.

Deinstitutionalization for Nick would never be an option in older models, as he'd probably never make it to one. Likewise, mainstreaming and inclusion are not a real concern, because the public school could never support his needs. If they tried, they wouldn't know where to start and when they did, they would introduce experiences that he would never be aware of. This example, in similar ways to the other children, would use great levels of public funding on models and systems that are not designed to address the needs of these children. They would then spend great levels of dollars to fund nursing care along with numerous additional staff and teachers trying everything in their cognitive arsenal to teach concepts. If by chance there were staff with advanced skill, they might attempt to implement sensory-based experiences, yet without the knowledge of the sequences necessary to produce consistent outcomes and without any skill to assess or evaluate the effectiveness of these approaches.

Having taken a closer look at the uniqueness of each client, planning can be accomplished more specifically and appropriately. Effects of mainstreaming, inclusion and institutionalization can be more clearly understood. This leads to a discussion of the IEP requirement of a least restrictive environment (LRE). The LRE is not a function of pre-existing systems or presumptions of centralized tradition, but rather should be an individualized designation for each child. For some it may be a more self-contained classroom wherein the environmental stimuli can be controlled for the nervous system of each child. This way we could avoid the looping phenomena that binds many people with disabilities in their repetitive behavior. Yet another scenario may be targeted inclusion, chosen for the specific achievements and development of that student. Finally, another child may best be suited for full inclusion to benefit from adapted academics and peer interaction.

This can be identified specifically for each student, child, or adult by carefully identifying and understanding the diagnosis. It is essential to identify what the diagnosis means related to processing and storage and recall of learned information and what stimuli set is most effective to achieve these ends. Additionally, a somewhat uncomfortable task is identifying the needed team members who are appropriately trained to treat the neurologic dysfunctions identified by the diagnosis as well as provide any functional standardized assessments needed for each child. For example, a child in level 1, 2 or 3 of sensory orientation training really would not need the services or expense of a special education professional; but rather more intensive interventions by a Neurologic Music Therapist (NMT), supported by neurologic trained physical therapists (PTs) and occupational therapists (OTs). Another scenario may not need a speech therapist as even pre-language skills are not the focus or need. In yet another situation, an NMT or neurologic trained PT or OT may not be needed as the disability may not have a neurologic foundation. I specify *neurologic* MT, PT and OT because traditionally educated therapists in these fields are not usually trained in the neural sequential model necessary for functional change. This model of targeted intervention and assessment is more effective and efficient financially for a system strapped for dollars and with poor outcomes.

I believe this is how the IEP was designed to be implemented, rather than from the perspective from tightly controlled bureaucrats who are always quick to implement tradition rather than the application of science.

Furthermore, consider for a moment the impact if we could also now begin to assign predictable funding costs and staffing patterns to each of these various functioning levels and reduce both the funding and staffing intensity as skills develop.

Chapter Four

The Neural Sequential Model

For decades academia has held to a model of education and learning based upon traditional methods that served us well for most of that history. Now, however, we are entering a new era of development due to several factors. First, we now raise and educate our children in environments that have little consistency and often include levels of toxic stress (Center on the Developing Child - Harvard University). Second, we have a greater knowledge base of how the brain works and how it responds to our current sensory environment.

Neurologic Music Therapy (NMT) is one such neural sequential model that addresses the fundamental issues produced by our hyper sensory communities. We must begin to understand the neurologic basis for disability and be bold to manage our children's environments to support healthy neurologic function. Even the typically developing infant needs this sequencing.

> *Who would begin exposing their newborn to high levels of motor activity and demanding or expecting verbal responses to even the ABC's?*

Then why do we expect the ABC's, verbal or pictorial, from our profoundly developmentally impaired four- or five- or even 21-year-old, when their brain is functioning like that of the infant?

Shouldn't we first assess whether they are attending, tracking stimuli or producing consistent motor activity to sensory stimulation?

Again, let us remember the following principles in rethinking early childhood and neurologic disabilities interventions.

A neurologic perspective through music perception structures:

1. Perception and production: Does the child consistently respond to external stimuli, including visual, auditory and tactile? Will he produce motor responses to interact with the external stimuli?

Each of the children highlighted in this book began in this phase of arousal and orientation to the environment. In the case of Andrew and Dan, we were able initially to facilitate motor responses to auditory and tactile stimuli. This initial motor activation produced motor activity sufficient to develop cortical connectivity in brain modules responsible for increasing levels of complexity of non-motor responses. Their specific diagnosis predicted more rapid development due to intact networks - Andrew, because his injury did not tear or shear brain matter, but instead produced swelling and hyper neurologic activity, and Dan, who likewise had to reorganize but needed patterns necessary to direct and wire predictable pathways of neural information. Thus, both children quickly oriented and began to produce age appropriate responses (chronologically appropriate, not developmentally appropriate). Andrew began responding with vocal sounds and Dan began by producing motor activity along with vocalizations. Both children produced these musical patterns on predefined sequences of rhythm and overlearned vocal patterns. The brain, once hearing or feeling a rhythm pattern, will always seek to complete that same pattern in future presentation of that pattern. Consider singing an ascending scale; do re mi fa so la ti ... and leaving off the final do? Every brain within earshot will complete that pattern, because that is what our cultural context does. Next time you attend a party, consider walking in a room of unknowing people and sing: "Shave and a haircut," and nothing else. Listen and see what happens. Consider why this is, in light of what we've discussed here.

Nick and Eric also required the input of patterned stimuli, both motor and auditory, to jumpstart the nervous system. Conversely, however, these boys were never going to begin responses at chronological levels because Nick had never learned them and Eric had the information erased from cortical regions, as exhibited by the scans showing no activity in correlated brain regions. Consequently, motor and auditory priming techniques facilitated developmental responses. Herein lies the remarkable results we achieved quickly in very early stages of neural-sensitive early childhood interventions.

2. Are they able to sustain attention to the environmental stimuli?

Phase two of our interventions for each of the four children looked again very similar. I planned for and achieved consistent and sustained quantity of response. With Andrew, we achieved increasing levels of first vocal and then verbal responses. Along with the vocalizations, the motor system began to respond with an increasing quantity of movement. His attempts to speak often were confused with very poor rate control, filled with stuttering and cluttering due to corresponding hyperactive and inconsistent neurologic activity. The consistent rhythm patterns and sequences instantly regulated and coordinated timing and rate control of vocal and motor patterns, piece by piece, as his internal control of initiation and sustaining of responses took over, enabling him to self-sustain attention or vigilance.

Dan in this phase is now engaged vocalizing and beginning to verbally sing along with the songs one at a time. By the end of most of them as I prep him to transfer to another song, he begins to hit his head and scream, consistently, every time. So, I back up and introduce a motor pattern with each song; asking for no singing other than what he chooses to self-initiate and that he will complete each song with the assigned motor activity, such as clapping for one melody and tapping toes for another. Amazingly but predictably with this model, he will complete several songs in succession while self-managing the song transitions with the motor actions. Finally, we re-introduce the vocalizations and he will now complete the entire pattern with vocal and motor activity. Once more

I then encouraged and introduced the words and he sang them too, entirely, and continued this way never ceasing, subsequently exploding into constant and consistent verbal communication with all staff and peers, in every situation and classroom environment.

Nick began with the movements with ascending and descending arms with the musical patterns, self-initiating these movements every time he heard the tune. More remarkably, within a week or so, he also began vocalizing on pitch with the ending of each musical phrase. This little interaction quickly expanded to immediate self-initiation of the vocalizations and a maintenance of them throughout each song phrase. Again, this is also sustaining of attention while purposefully engaging in the environmentally appropriate experience.

Eric also exhibited the sustained response to stimuli, first by motor and then by vocal engagement. He first began wildly batting and swinging at musical instruments as they were presented before him. He also began bouncing and rocking intensely in his chair every time music began or when he recognized a staff member coming in and talking with him or near him. Staff of course was very concerned about his "negative behavior" that they quickly wanted to extinguish, but I'll raise here the question I also raised to them. Is it a negative behavior because it looks like one from the neural typical person, or is he merely producing his first excited response to the world he desperately wants to know, learn about and interact with, but he has no internal control to initiate or inhibit motor activity? Furthermore, isn't uncontrolled movement the first kind of movement we see or realize with initial development of a newborn? Second, don't we then begin working with the newborn to gradually develop motor control that leads to holding, banging objects together, scooting, crawling, rolling, sitting up, pulling up to stand, etc.?

3. Is the child able to switch his/her attention from one item to another? Will he consistently alternate between competing issues in the environment? Can he maintain attention to a prescribed task while competing issues are occurring in the environment?

Here we are now in another stage for each of our children: higher levels of attention, divided and alternating. In the case of Eric and Nick, this isn't even a factor because as we stand in our neural sensitive process, neither of them has reached this level of functioning. As a result, it is not necessary to introduce these two specific and structured interventions, and if we tried the result would most likely not be positive. Both Eric and Nick are desperately trying to develop sensory control to sustain attention and continue the prolonged responses in keeping with the environmental factors. Dan and Andrew, on the other hand, have achieved neurologic control of alternating and dividing their own attention. These functions were achieved by producing a music sequence that facilitated specific motor actions. Dan, as earlier noted, accomplished sensory motor skill to march with the rhythmic cue of "When the Saints Go Marching In." He also then learned to sway or rock left, right and back, rocking with another tune. When the tunes are combined into one composition, he automatically alternates his actions, and then attention, based upon the auditory and rhythmic cues. This then immediately translated into his ability to shift and change from one school lesson to the next, and from one nursing intervention or therapy to the next, with complete absence of head slapping or screaming, which had been incorrectly labeled a negative behavior.

The next step for Dan included encouraging him to initiate and maintain his motor actions when the musical sequence was introduced, meanwhile, myself or other staff and children performed a completely different song and dance or even simply his own, but 180 degrees out of phase.

These accomplishments, of course, have much broader implications than simply his skill. Remember, if he can now not only attend, learn current content, block out other activities in his environment, and functionally switch between multiple stations in his classroom, then he really doesn't need all the extra special education or attention.

Andrew is another case of rapid success using these specific neurologic techniques. Once he began responding and maintaining attention control, vigilance over time, we used similar alternating and divided musical neural stimuli to accelerate executive functions. In Andrew's situation, restorative rather than developmental, his ability to achieve these levels of attention came almost automatically with very little specific intervention, but simple practice. This would resemble a learning process of a typically developing kid. Circle time in the mostly younger group of kids is now almost led completely by him. The special education staff enters and asks generally, "What's first," and Andrew begins the name song and selects and sings to each child in the room after the teacher begins to spell each child's name. Andrew interrupts, finishes spelling the name and then sings hello to each. Meanwhile, multiple competing stimuli continue in the classroom with nurse conversation and interventions occurring all around him.

4. While attending to any prescribed task, can the child produce or identify meaningful perception of pitch, tempo, or patterns of rhythm?

5. Does the child sing recognizable melodies, patterns or lyric phrases? Can the child articulate a song verse or create his/her own phrase with meaning and context?

6. Is articulation of any of the verbal music production clear, understandable, and within the tempo of normal singing?

These next few concepts bring in a whole new thought process. Each of the children examined in this book reached musical milestones more quickly than non-musical ones. We can understand the renewed musical skill of Andrew, but Dan's quick musical development is a testament to the power of music and rhythm to facilitate that immediate change in the brain, despite the missing hippocampus. Even before the advanced motor and communication explosion, Dan began vocalizing with accurate rhythm and pitch. In addition, even more remarkable is the rhythmic and vocal development of Eric. With the virtual re-do, he first self-engaged with rhythmic bouncing and vocalizations of expression and excitement. How vital it is to be able to recognize each of these very specific responses in light of the specific diagnosis and neurologic based developmental understanding. Any random application of rhythmic and musical intervention would have produced a similar random and unpredictable myriad of responses. Often in common practice today, each of these random responses are applauded as development, but most often never consistently realized again. This perpetual pattern has been the sad story of developing adults and school children alike for decades.

Treatment methods:

1. How do we select appropriate music experiences to meet a child wherever he functions within the hierarchy previously listed?
2. Are we careful and patient enough to understand the underlying brain dysfunction and apply standardized approaches to facilitate change?
3. Despite traditions and social pressure, are we clinically confident and educated enough to implement a protocol necessary to foster meaningful change?

Chapter Five

Taking on the Money Monkey!

An underlying factor in solving these issues plaguing our system and children is of course the money.

Is there enough? How do we allocate these funds? Even more challenging is who holds the purse?

In Wisconsin, we have begun looking at and tackling these very issues through the roll out of our Family Care managed care model. Simply put, care management organizations apply and bid for contracts to provide specific services in a specific region and families and/or guardians select to participate in one specific organization. They are then assigned or choose a care manager who is responsible for educating the consumer or their family as to the options of service available. A good step in the right direction, but a key piece that is still working itself out is how and who is to educate case managers and families what the best practices are and if cutting edge options are available. A couple of issues are important to point out for our consideration.

Costs: long-term, short-term, special education, and rehabilitation.

Let's begin by taking a closer look at some fiscal data from Wisconsin's Department of Health Services and the Department of Public Instruction.

I'll begin at the early childhood and special education process. The most recent data shows that we spend approximately $1.5 billion per year with a total of 121,000 students. Of these students about 3,800 are severe profound. Average per pupil spending is about $11,500 a year. Most children of the 121,000 have mild disabilities or are learning disabled receiving speech language, reading support, etc. and use very limited funds, while the 3,800 students with severe and profound disabilities consume closer to $25,000 each or $95,000,000 per year (data from Wisconsin Department of Public Instruction).

Much of this funding is spent on the overhead of special education and support services to foster adaptations for inclusion. When these students complete schooling, typically around age 21, most have not made measurable progress toward functional independence. Then they are kept at home or in community-based facilities and receive home-based care and attend day activity programs where they are exposed to community inclusion that includes bus rides to festivals, fairs and zoos. I exaggerate a bit, but the result isn't far from the description. The virtual warehousing results in perpetual illness, a drain on our health care system, behavioral and emotional outbursts, a drain on our mental health system, and genuinely unfulfilled lives. The final result in my opinion is simply not acceptable since I have described that there are alternatives.

In many cases these precious people have been so trained or "reinforced" that they are unable to think, choose or express themselves. They have been exposed to various and numerous experiential curricula designed to enhance and develop cognitive and social skills. Each of these goals is higher, more volitional cognitive function. As we've discussed, these milestones are only truly achieved after fundamental neurological sequences have been laid. Examples from our caseload include careful assessment of where they fall in our hierarchy: MSOT level I, II, or III (arousal, orientation, or vigilance). Second, are they able to initiate and maintain attention in order to learn cognitive content? Is the motor and cognitive activity consistent, time ordered and sequenced in organized patterns? The well-meaning staff that have cared for them have used behavior methods to produce meaningless responses to the world without loving, caring natural supports that you and I need and thrive on. By this, I mean a family that cares, and doing a job that they love, or a community church that really loves them, respects them for who they are created to be and desires to serve one another in love.

Applied Behavioral Analysis

Historical context

The Enlightenment, the Great Awakening, and the Industrial Revolution are all advances in human society that began to perpetuate knowledge pursuit and the inquiry into the mind of mankind. In 1913 John Watson, one such pioneer, took a shot at describing or explaining the reason for human behavior. His theory was based on the observation of human behavior and thus his explanations were based upon pure application and understanding of those human responses. Watson postulated that people will naturally explore the world and these explorations will naturally be reinforced or punished based upon the natural result of interaction with the world. If the response to an inquiry is met with a positive reinforcer, that inquiry will continue. If an inquiry is met with an unpleasant result, that behavior will most likely cease. This theory presumes individuals can and will respond to their environment.

A few years later, well-known B. F. Skinner (1953) introduced a systematic application of the behavioral theory as it relates to the following concepts. First, reinforcement, that when an action is met with a pleasing response, the behavior will increase and continue. When the behavior is met with a response that isn't so pleasant, an individual will most likely not continue that particular action. Once these basic behavioral responses are learned, they can be shaped through prompting and then the assistance will be faded away until no longer necessary. Skinnerian theory is possibly most well-known for the rats and the levers pushed for food or learning the quickest way to get through the maze and find the food.

Some years later yet again, Lovaas (1987) introduced his method, most commonly used with autism spectrum disorders (ASD). His approach took off and is still used commonly, with modifications, for today's ASD populations. An unfortunate aspect of his approach was the use of aversive stimuli; meaning that the natural result of some activities would be an unpleasant natural consequence. Some examples may include pain, accidents, social isolation, etc.

Today, a blending and almost unrecognizable application of each of these is used and accepted as correct, normal, and necessary for our system to support the most vulnerable in our communities. Unfortunately, the results continue to be poor and ineffective in fostering true independence and meaningful inclusion in our communities. As we look at these models considering our case examples, when we understand individual diagnostic differentiation, we can begin to understand what works, what doesn't, and why.

While keeping these basic principles of neuroscience in mind, we can begin to understand the need for change in our early childhood environments. This shift will better serve the neurologic needs of these fragile children. A key step in the right direction, however, puts a wrench in the spinning gears of a failing public education system that appears to support tradition and tenure over scientific best practice. Perhaps this renaissance of knowledge can begin to untangle the politically correct mantra of the year. If environments must be structured to support the cognitive health of these children, then we need to rethink the one-size-fits-all model of modern inclusion. Research-based, clinical intellect should guide parents and families to choose the model best fitting their own child. Likewise, communities and systems must support the choices of the families. Private sector solutions should and will arrive and compete through best practice to provide the most effective treatment. Political systems must be reformed and education would be based upon science. Those blinded by policy will finally fall to the heap of failed approaches. Our children will be the beneficiaries of this carefully planned inheritance.

Conclusions

Environmental Implications

A first key step to foster positive change considers the environmental support and structures that are effective and appropriate for the children. Accurately assessed and then treated children make significant developmental gains. These gains, when tracked and measured, can guide a care team to choose integration options appropriate for each child.

For example, in the case of Andrew, staffing and clinical methods would focus on recovery, rather than educational goals. When his initial goals were met, that team membership would be reassessed and reorganized to include educators and skill development experts that would continue the push toward independence.

Phase one of Andrew's treatment might cost $2,000 per month, but then quickly move to $1,000 per month in line with our state's current expense for a child enrolled in the statewide special needs voucher program. In this way, for each consumer in care, cost will reduce quickly as skills develop. Educational systems need to be flexible enough to support the targeted inclusion of these children to advance the positive trajectory of development. That means being flexible enough to continuously shift and modify both the service team, the treatment setting and financial resources. State officials must return the power of education to the families and local teams, thus respecting the will and choices they make. This is in keeping with the spirit and letter of the Individualized Education Plan.

Developmental and training implications

In the current system, the children have been left behind with the false promise of a quality and free education. Looking at the amounts spent, and the outcome data, it has been neither free nor equal. Evidence to this end is the less than 50 percent graduation rate in my own community. Educators are expected to dutifully follow the methods of University silos filled with academics designed to destroy intellect and solidify an ever-changing goal post of relativism, today's new religion. Classrooms in my own experience devolve into chaos daily with educators ill-trained to address the neurologic disabilities spawned from similarly chaotic communities. Foundational principles of a community centered with a spiritual conviction have been stripped by leaders striving to eliminate the one thing that held ancient and recent cultures together - that is a spiritually centered bio-psychosocial culture. Parents and families must be centered and supported by these foundational principles lest their liberty and very core be stripped by egalitarianists poised to secure a false welfare over them.

Fiscal policy implications

Our current system has clearly failed when less than 50 percent of students graduate and those that do are not prepared to secure or create the jobs to support their families, not to mention the debt this current generation has amassed. The current system is expensive, and the product is subpar. By embracing the principles delineated in this book, we can dramatically improve the fiscal outlook for state and local government. A clinically informed model, rather than continuous increases in funding for traditional public education, would provide a model wherein funding can be reduced as meaningful development improves. Initially, more trained personnel would be necessary to support the needs of the severely impaired; however, as rehabilitative or developmental gains are made, less restrictive environments will be utilized along with less specialized staff with lower costs associated with them. As mentioned earlier, initial phases may cost around $2,000 a month, but quickly reduce to around $1,000 a month, by using staff and methods appropriate for each child. More children will quickly meet levels of independence that reduce the long-term care costs associated with current disability populations. If children leave the school system as "super utilizers" of state support funds, they continue to use them with increasing intensity for a lifetime. If children finish school with increased cognitive, motor and communication skills, they also finish proud with increased independence. Here is the framework for the first Developmental Reimbursement Reduction Model (DRRM) that I have developed. Looking at the neural sequential model I have discussed will, through data, identify for each diagnosis what service may be needed. Furthermore, this data-driven approach will identify what staff will be needed to facilitate that progress. These specific costs and developed skills can be directly tied to scores on standardized assessments that identify what neurologic process must be addressed first; what staff should be utilized in that step and reasonably predict what the next phase for each child will look like. This will be based purely on assessment data and statistics gathered across the system comparing similar diagnostic categories. Additionally, I will unveil to legislators and education leaders a saving model much like the one we introduced in Wisconsin with our medical assistance purchase plan, called a Lifestyles Savings Plan. This savings model will enable individuals with special needs, or their families and guardians, to put money aside tax-free in a way that would not affect eligibility for Medicaid insurance. Families, loved ones, or anybody else could contribute to the trust that would be used, managed, and owned by individuals. Currently, the assets held by an individual's family are counted against them in determining eligibility for additional services and financial support. If significant resources can be held in trust for each person, and used according to self-determined needs, then each family holds the power and control of what is needed and/or chosen by free will and expert advice. We tend to spend wisely when the risk of running out is facing our every decision. Isn't this a more truthful example of the least restrictive environment (LRE)?

Imagine with me for a moment. Join me in remembering the words of John Lennon. "Imagine all the lonely people." Imagine the lonely children. Must we accept this state of loneliness, knowing what we know? I must separate from

John Lennon on the other points: imagining a world without religion and without countries. If we continue to eliminate or allow the elimination of borders and countries, we are left with a few ruling all the people and establishing for us all what is good, right, and appropriate. Where we see these patterns today leaves us with public school and human service programs solidifying hopelessness. I cannot imagine how the least of these would fare with no religion and no more countries. I cannot imagine that resulting in Andrew talking, Dan walking, and Eric squealing with joy from new discoveries of life. Please join me in harnessing the power of music to continue restoring sight to the blind, enabling the lame to walk, and the mute to talk.

Additional Resources

If you need help, or want more information to improve your or someone else's situation, please reach out to one of the following resources.

1. Your local aging and disability resource center
2. Local case management or assessment resources, including functional screenings
3. JohnDaubert.com
4. Accelerate-ability-llc.com
5. https://www.linkedin.com/in/johnhartmanmke/
6. Linkedin@JohnDHartman.com
7. https://nmtacademy.co/

References

Balasubramani, P. P., & Hayden, B. (2018). Orbitofrontal neuron ensembles contribute to inhibitory control. *Biorxiv, the Reprint Server for Biology.* doi: https://doi.org/10.1101/452938

Bradt J, & Dileo C. (2009). Music for stress and anxiety reduction in coronary heart disease patients. *Cochrane Database of Systematic Reviews, 2,* doi:10.1002/14651858.CD006577.pub2.

Bradt, J. Dileo, C, & Shim, M. (2013). Music interventions for preoperative anxiety. *Cochrane Systematic Review - Intervention Version*

Curtis, W. J., & Nelson, C. A. (2003). Toward building a better brain: Neurobehavioral outcomes, mechanisms, and processes of environmental enrichment. In S. S. Luthar (Ed.), *Resilience and vulnerability: Adaptation in the context of childhood adversities* (pp. 463-488). New York, NY, US: Cambridge University Press. http://dx.doi.org/10.1017/CBO9780511615788.021

Dozza, M., Chiari, L., & Horak, F. B. (2005). Audio-biofeedback improves balance in patients with bilateral vestibular loss. *Archives of Physical Medicine and Rehabilitation, 86*(7), 1401-3.

Dozza, M., Chiari, L., Hlavacka, F., Cappello, A., & Horak, F. B. (2006). Effects of linear versus sigmoid coding of visual or audio biofeedback for the control of upright stance. *IEEE Transactions on Neural Systems & Rehabilitation Engineering, 14*(4), 505-512.

Effenberg, A. O., & Mechling, H. (1998). Bewegung hörbar machen–Warum? *Zur Perspektive einer systematischen Umsetzung von Bewegung in Klänge. psychologie und sport, 1,* 29-38.

Graham, J. (2004). Communication with the uncommu nicative: Music therapy with pre-verbal adults. *British Journal of Learning Disabilities, 32*(1), 24-29.

Grandin, T. (1992). Calming effects of deep touch pressure in patients with autistic disorder, college students, and animals. *Journal of Child and Adolescent Psychopharmacology, 2* (1), 63-72.

Guldenmund, P., Stender, J., & Heine, L. (2012). Mindsight: Diagnostics in disorders of consciousness. *Critical Care Research and Practice*, Article ID 624724, 13 pages http://dx.doi.org/10.1155/2012/624724

Hyland, S. (2018). Optimizing neurological development learning difficulty, immature development of primitive & postural reflexes. 8/25/18 http://suehyland.co.uk/ ond/primitive-reflexes/?doing_wp_cron=1535208660. 4594190120697021484375

Jeong, S., & Kim, M. T. (2007). Effects of a theory-driven music and movement program for stroke survivors in a community setting. *Applied Nursing Research, 20*(3), 125-131.

Kübler, A., Furdea, A., Halder, S., Hammer, E. M., Nijboer, F., & Kotchoubey, B. (2009). A brain-computer interface controlled auditory event-related potential P300 spelling system for locked-in patients. *Annals of the New York Academy of Sciences, 1157*(1), 90-100.

Kübler, A., & Neumann, N. (2005). Brain-computer interfaces: The key for the conscious brain locked into a paralyzed body. *Progress in Brain Research, 150*, 513-525.

Luft, A.R., McCombe-Waller, S., Whitall, J., Forrester, L.W., Macko, R., Sorkin, J. D., Schulz, J. B., Goldberg, A. P., & Hanley, D. F. (2004). Repetitive bilateral arm training and motor cortex activation in chronic stroke: A randomized controlled trial. *Journal of the American Medical Association, 292*(15), 1853-1861.

Lovass, O. (1987). Behavioral treatment and normal educational and intellectual functioning in young autistic children. *Journal of Consulting and Clinical Psychology, 55*, 3-9.

Magee, W. L. (2007). Music as a diagnostic tool in low awareness states: Considering limbic responses. *Brain Injury, 21*, 593-599.

McCombe, W.S. & Whitall, J. (2005). Hand dominance and side of stroke affect rehabilitation in chronic stroke. *Clinical Rehabilitation, 19*(5), 544-551.

McCombe Waller, S. & Whitall, J. (2006). Combining bilateral and distal arm training to promote arm and hand recovery in patients with chronic hemiparesis: A case report. *Proceedings of the 4th World Congress for Neurorehabilitation*, 2-80.

McEachin, J. J., Smith, T., & Lovaas, O. I. (1993). Long-term outcome for children with autism who received early intensive behavioral treatment. *American Journal on Mental Retardation, 97* (4), 359-372.

Noda, R., Maeda, Y., & Yoshino, A. (2004). Therapeutic time window for musicokinetic therapy in a persistent vegetative state after severe brain damage. *Brain Injury, 18*(5), 509-515.

Owen, A. M., & Coleman, M. (2008). Functional imaging in the vegetative state. *Nature Reviews Neuroscience, 9*, 235-243.

Pacchetti, C., Aglieri, R., Mancini, F., Martignoni, E., & Nappi, G. (1998). Active music therapy and Parkinson's disease: Methods. *Functional Neurology, 13*(1), 57-67.

Pacchetti, C., Mancini, F., Aglieri, R., Fundarò, C., Martignoni, E., & Nappi, G. (2000). Active music therapy in Parkinson's disease: an integrative method for motor and emotional rehabilitation. *Psychosomatic Medicine, 62*(3), 386-393.

Petacchi, A., Laird, A. R., Fox, P. T., & Bower, J. M. (2005). Cerebellum and auditory function: An ALE meta-analysis of functional neuroimaging studies. *Human Brain Mapping, 25*(1), 118-128.

Purdie, H. (1997). Music therapy in neurorehabilitation: Recent developments and new challenges. *Critical Reviews in Physical and Rehabilitation Medicine, 9*(3-4), 205-21.

Sacks, O. (1998). Music and the brain. In C.M. Tomaino (Ed.), *Clinical applications of music in neurologic rehabilitation* (pp. 1-18). St. Louis, MO: MMB Music, Inc.

Skinner, B. F. (1953). *The possibility of a science of human behavior.* NY: The Free House.

Thaut, M. H. (2005). *Rhythm, Music, and the Brain: Scientific Foundations and Clinical Applications.* New York: Taylor & Francis.

Thaut, M. H. (2015). Neurobiological foundations of neurologic music therapy: Rhythmic entrainment and the motor system. *Frontiers in Psychology, 6*. 10.3389/fpsyg.2014.01185.

Torres, E. B, Donnellan, A. M. (16 March, 2015). Autism the movement perspective. *Frontiers in Integrative Neuroscience.* https://doi.org/10.3389/fnint.2015.00012

Voss, H. U., Uluğ, A. M., Dyke, J. P., Watts, R., Kobylarz, E. J., McCandliss, B. D., et al., (2006). Possible axonal regrowth in late recovery from the minimally conscious state. *Journal of Clinical Investigation, 116*, 2005–2011. doi: 10.1172/JCI27021

Watson, John B. (1930). *Behaviorism* (revised edition). Chicago: University of Chicago Press.

Whitall, J., McCombe, Waller, S., Silver, K. H., & Macko, R. F. (2000). Repetitive bilateral arm training with rhythmic auditory cueing improves motor function in chronic hemiparetic stroke. *Stroke, 31*(10), 2390-2395.

Yasuhara, A., & Sugiyama, Y. (2001). Music therapy for children with Rett syndrome. *Brain and Development, 23*(Suppl. 1), S82-S84.

Zasler, N. D. (1999). Ask the doctor. *Brain Injury Source, 3*(3), 47.

Printed in the United States
By Bookmasters